Splinterbone

Splinterbone

◆

Making Peace
With the Pain of Arthritis

Laura Folk

iUniverse, Inc.
New York Lincoln Shanghai

Splinterbone
Making Peace With the Pain of Arthritis

iUniverse, Inc.

For information address:
iUniverse, Inc.
2021 Pine Lake Road, Suite 100
Lincoln, NE 68512
www.iuniverse.com

ISBN: 0-595-31647-6

Printed in the United States of America

For my mother,
Eleanor Frank,
God Never Made a Greener Thumb!

Contents

Acknowledgements

I would like to thank my family in advance for understanding my need to write this book, as they do not yet know about it. I also would like to thank Lisa for dealing with my pain; I know it is not easy at times. Finally, I would like to extend thanks to all the doctors who have tried to help me, for in the end, they are committed to ending suffering, even if the methods are at times fruitless.

Preface

This book was written with the intention to help all those people that suffer from the disease of osteoarthritis, but especially for women. This is not because men do not suffer from the disease, but because I am a woman and do not have the insight of a male perspective. This can be a very lonely disease, and I hope that by reading my journal you realize you are not alone, and can be your own best friend on a daily basis. This book was also written as a tribute to my mother and to all mothers that have lived a challenging life. While some aspects of tribulation may not be pretty, they are the cornerstone of character, and should be remembered as such. For those of you who still have your mother, I suggest you take the time to get to know her as an individual, and heal your rifts before they become bone deep.

Because this is a true journal, the material may seem to wander and ramble at times, often shifting focus. This is a natural process for journal writing as anyone that has kept a journal over a long period of time knows. I have been journal writing since I was fourteen years old. I have stayed true to the journal form for a reason. It is hard to stay focused when dealing with intense pain on a daily basis .The emotional states that accompany ongoing pain are also debilitating. In order to go on with one's life, one has to consciously learn to start over every day, no matter what happened the day before. If experiencing this through reading this book is disconcerting, then I have done my job well, for then you will know what it is like to attempt to maintain focus on moving forward in one's life while under duress.

In the journal journey, I relive past adventures, connect with nature, and find new connections to my mother's family. These experiences are a spontaneous part of the journaling process. The importance of being spontaneous when using writing as a healing tool cannot be overstated. This book was a healing tool for me, and I share it with you as an example of the actual process. I have inserted meditations along the way as a supplement to the journal. I encourage you to start your own journal, and to create your own meditations. My story is merely a jumping off point. You have your own story to tell, and your own adventures to live.

This piece is short, and some may think it is missing what is called meat and potatoes. Whatever it may or may not be missing, it is my experience, and I have shared it with you because I want to make your life better, easier, and freer from pain. I hope it inspires you to face your pain and embrace it. This book is not fluffy; it tells it like it is. It represents the true nature of the splinterbone woman. Maybe you are one, maybe you are not. Maybe you want to be one, maybe you don't. Whatever you are, and whatever you strive to be, it is my sincere wish that you be it and do it because you have made peace with your pain.

Remembering (Anniversary of My Mother's Death)

Smooth and jagged, white with grey flecks, curved in places. This is the splinter of bone that lies in the tin box that holds my mother's remains. Smooth and jagged, this describes it all—her life, her sufferings, her personality and the disease she passed down to me ~ "Arthur" as she called it ~ Arthritis.

February 13 was the 2nd year anniversary of my mother's death. That was two days ago. It was also the same day I had the pleasure of finding out I have the same bone splintering disease as my mother. Why do I call it bone splintering? Because that is what it does, it cracks your ease into a million pieces of jagged pain, crushing pain, a crucible of pain. It takes the backbone of your life, your strength, and stability and breaks you, making you an emotional mess.

The funny thing is this is also what watching my mother die did to me. It broke me apart, spilled out all the unmet needs, and shattered my makeshift personality. I tried so hard to not be like my mother, yet, two years later to the day; I am finding that at the deepest level, in my very bones, I am created in her image.

What a revelation; she rises from the ashes every time I rise from bed with burning hips, swollen fingers, and screaming toes. I tried so hard not to be my mother. Not to be negative, tactless, and long-suffering. Only now do I know she lived on cut glass for almost half her life. I have bartered with myself for years; am I a hero, a wretch, a Nazi, a product of a crazy grandmother? The smooth and the jagged; I wanted her to be smooth, a genteel lady, a cultured pearl, a 3-piece suit. Wow, that is what I have tried to be. Guess what? I'm not. No, I am a splinterbone, a woman hewn from the genetic pool, carved by striving to be different.

So this love/hate relationship with my mother has also been one with me, only I blamed that on her too. They say you will understand what your mother went through when you have a child of your own. The day I found out about the arthritic spurs on my spine, I said to myself, "I can, for the first time, say I'm glad I did not have any kids so they don't have to suffer this genetic nightmare." Well I have always wanted children so this was a strong statement. But now, I see that this disease is like the child I never had. It is the creature that reflects my mothers' trials. I have had an intellectual understanding of her pain and grief, but until now have not really understood anything.

This bone child, this splintering pain, is the closest thing I have to a connection with my mother. I watched her breath leave her body, saw her wince two times and felt the last electrical tremble in her arm before her body turned stone cold. There were no last words as she was incoherent when I arrived at the hospital that afternoon, not that she would have known who I was anyway due to her Alzheimer's, so I did not get to say goodbye. I have tried to make peace with her for the last 15 years, but the rift was bone deep. How could I make peace with someone I rejected so deeply yet needed and wanted just as much, again a reflection of her? You see, I never accepted the creature she was, carved from her father and sisters' early deaths, her mothers attempt to murder her and final suicide leaving her an orphan with all hopes dashed.

I have never really appreciated the woman my mother was, although I have tried to convince myself that I have. Hence, I have never appreciated the woman I am. My loathing of her and my self-loathing has been one and the same. I did not know this until this moment. It has taken the birth of my bone child Arthur (itis), to realize this. His labor has been long. Now what do I do with a screaming child whose very nature is pain?

The Peace That Comes
(With Feeling the Pain)

Pain brings choice. You either let it overtake you like a pack of wolves on the hunt, or you sit still in the middle of it and ride like a surfer. Some waves are ripples on the surface; others are like the 50-year storm wave Kurt Russell waited for in the movie *Point Break*. Either way, you rest on top of the experience and wait, mindful of the medium. In surfing it is water, wind, the ebb and flow of the tide. With pain it is more like the pitch of sound. Sometimes it is high and piercing, sometimes low and rumbling, but there is always white noise.

I do not know how my mother coped with her pain. I could say she did it with Budweiser, Kools, and her green thumb, but I would be only partially correct. Now that I feel like I know my mother better than ever in sharing her pain, I realize I did not know her at all, in the sense that I cannot presume what she thought or felt, or how she really coped. This view restores dignity to her, and to me. In the mystery of not knowing I free her to be an intelligent survivor of her lot in life, instead of the helpless woman gasping for breath on her deathbed.

All my opinions of her past shortcomings melt into that realization, and become a rebirth. A new relationship is born. I have felt like I missed out on any relationship with my mother, and that since she was reduced to a pile of ash on my altar, that it was impossible to have any kind of contact. Yet, here I sit with a totally unexpected, untried for situation. For two years I have attempted to make peace with her death. I planted some of her ashes in a ponytail palm tree, and inserted a picture of her in the container. I expected this to bring peace as she loved her plants so. To my surprise this did not shorten the distance between us. Of course I take care of the plant, and call it mom, and now I realize it was like our old relationship—a mental exercise, not an organic one.

In feeling the pain my mother wrought on me by birth, I sense her presence throughout my whole being. I always thought when my mother died I would be haunted by her. In freeing her from my opinion I have brought her back to me, to the place I lost her in the first place. From the time I can remember there was distance between us, an emotional void. I wanted her love so desperately, to be held, acknowledged. My whole life I sought it, and until now, never received it.

Others have told me that of course my mother loved me no matter what I thought, and I tried to convince myself of that intellectually, but I never really felt it or believed it, I only felt the longing ~ it consumed me. My whole life has been an experience of bouncing between rejecting her, to try and find me, and being burned in the self-destructive fires of wanting to merge with the mother love I never felt. If this sounds exhausting, well no wonder I feel burned out. You could say how sad it is only now you realize your mother loved you. But it is not sad at all. It is not happy either. It is just an all pervading truth, one that will sustain me as I ride the waves of physical pain. My mother did not love me sweetly; she loved me bone deep, like a splinterbone, like a leg that has been broken with the marrow oozing out. This is what it was, this is who she was, and to accept someone for who they are is true love. I did not feel she ever accepted me, but then again I am assuming I knew all her thoughts. I cannot rob my mother of her path of realization in life, or death, by presumption. She has passed over to a new adventure, and in some form continues on. Now I can let her go because I know she has the tools to do so freed from my image of her. I have her strength and her rugged razor-sharp bite on life. I also have the sensitivity that screams when the marrow leaks out. The thing is, now I know I got that from her too, not in spite of her like I once thought.

The peace that comes in being with ones pain is the only real salve for the wound. It is the cure, the way out of hell.

Meditation on Pain

Now I am going to ask you to do something that you might not want to do. I am going to ask you to actually focus on the pain you are feeling right now. If you are not feeling pain at this moment, then you will be asked to bring to mind the last time you were in severe pain. Do not be afraid of this exercise. The purpose is not to make the pain greater, or to make it go totally away. The purpose is to be with the pain, to accept it, and at the same time to not be attached to it. Perhaps you have done similar exercises or meditations.

Sit in a comfortable position. I am not going to ask you to close your eyes because you will not be able to read this if you do. Most books tell you to close your eyes and imagine this or that. Unless you have the meditation tape recorded, it is hard to read, practice the instructions, and read some more. Just relax and take some slow deep breaths. Now, as you are reading these words, I want you to allow yourself to feel the pain wherever it is. As you breathe in imagine the pain going up through your nose as a dark cloud. As you take it in to your lungs imagine a bright, white, clean receptacle in your lungs, kind of like a bottle. Let the smoke go into the bottle.

When all the smoke enters into the bottle it is transformed into a healing balm of whatever color you wish to make it. Now, on your out breath imagine this mixture comes out of your nose and flows over and through the painful area. Do this exercise for about ten minutes. When you have finished begin reading the next paragraph.

If you are still feeling pain it is okay, remember I said the purpose was not to make the pain go away. Do you feel a sense of love and caring for yourself? If you do, it is compassion coming forth from that part of you that is detached from the pain. You can call this aspect of yourself whatever you want. Being compassionate to yourself will allow you to heal your relationship with yourself. You have a better chance of healing your body when you are in balance with mind and emotion. Finding this balance will be easier if you feel love and compassion for yourself and your pain, instead of fighting and resisting it.

I encourage you to practice this exercise for awhile. If it becomes familiar, eventually you may automatically begin to feel compassion for yourself the moment your pain is evident. This could have the effect of lessening the pain, or at least making it easier to cope with. Feel free to change the images you use in the meditation. Be creative and follow your intuition. I have allowed some space on this page for you to write in any ideas that may have come to you while doing this exercise so you can use them the next time you practice.

_____

_____

_____

_____

_____

_____

_____

_____

_____

_____

_____

_____

_____

_____

_____

_____

_____

_____

_____

_____

The Habit of Time
(Coping Day to Day)

Almost two weeks have passed since the diagnosis of my plight, and while I have a new and enduring appreciation for my mother; the changing face of this malady hits hard. The habit of caving into fear is strong and time plays tricks on the lessons learned.

Moments of revelation are a natural painkiller, but that's just it; they are moments. They cannot be bottled up like a pharmaceutical prescription and doled out times X. Revelation is a miracle that jettisons one forward in the game, but if you are not careful habit can land on you, and send you back two moves. The only real prescription for keeping the momentum is to create a new habit, one more in line with the fabric of the revelation itself.

In meeting my mother inside myself I cannot play the daily game in the same way, or I am doomed to fall prey as the dis-ease progresses. I must make a habit of remembering that I found peace, and leave a space open for more to enter. I cannot recreate the revelation I had two weeks ago. As an organic experience it has already assimilated itself, and changed form. I also cannot sit, and wait for another to come, or try to force it. All I can do is start fresh every day, and practice making peace with my pain as it changes in unexpected ways. It is tempting to expect liberation after clarity. Expectation is merely another habit, and a dangerous one.

What I am proposing is not really creating another habit; it is more like making a choice every day to sit with the moment whatever it brings. Be with the morning light, the delight of free movement, and the twist of the neck two minutes later that brings fear of surgery. Here enters projection, the cohort of fear. It is beginning to sound like an exhausting game of guarding oneself. Pain is exhausting; fear is exhausting and most of all the expectation of more pain born of projection.

Stop   leave space for   Peace   to enter. Ride the current wave for what it is right now. I cannot escape from my body, or the stressful job that gets increasingly harder to perform. I can however take note that I am not the pain, or the job, and in that space decide to enjoy this organic moment to its fullest.

March 1st
(Two Weeks Later)

I hear drummers in the distance; the Annual Native American Pow Wow is in town. They are dancing to the heartbeat of the drum. I used to be much closer to that culture which is part of my heritage. Healing was my passion. Finding the root of any problem, digging in the dirt of despair, and pulling out the cause, I find myself stripped of this passion now. It is like an ax that has gone dull from lack of maintenance. My sharpening stone is sitting on the shelf of lost vision. Perhaps I am just depressed from the pain, or the financial stresses of my predicament. Arguments with loved ones are easier now also. That space containing peace is hard to keep open.

The brave warrior has lost her paint. The dreamer, the planner, all the things I have been seem to crumble beneath the constant burning, the striving to be strong for others, and to carry on as usual. I am at a loss for direction, for a great idea to rescue me from the fallen city of my dreams. In plain English, I have to redefine myself and my capabilities again. This lurching toward old age and death is a real bummer.

April 18th
(Six Weeks Wandering)

Preliminary tests show osteoarthritis changes. I have an appointment with the bone doctor next month. The warming weather has helped the symptoms, although my fat body is weighing heavy on problem joints. Medicines sit on the shelf, sometimes they help, and sometimes not. I can understand my mother's beer drinking in light of this experience. However, I choose sobriety. I feel myself gearing up to creative expression of some sort. I have been coloring Mandalas, and find it relaxing.

I want to live simpler. I crave ease. In preparing my will, and other papers, there is a calm acceptance of this impermanent life. I started with gusto, and clinging, planning so many details to be remembered. Now I just fill out the papers to cover the basics with the important things being considered. If this all sounds drab and colorless, I apologize. The balance between my changing body and the beat of the industrial drum is precarious. I have ideas for a new business. I don't want to feel old, and at the end of productivity, and yet I'd love to swing in a hammock and just be pain free. Rambling, yes I know. Where is this piece of writing taking me, and you? Will it be a book, another exercise or a script for a new idea? Will it sit in the computer or will it evolve and actually help someone find new hope?

Meditation on Depression

It should be evident from reading the past couple of passages that I am depressed. Pain does that. I am sure you could tell me all kinds of stories about what pain has done to you and I am going to give you the space and time to do that in just a little while. Right now I want to do a similar exercise with depression that we did with pain. Again, feeling depressed is not something you like to experience or re-experience; however, learning to feel those intense emotions and not be swallowed up by them is a valuable tool.

Again, I am going to ask you to sit comfortably and read while you practice the exercise. You may or may not be depressed right now, although reading my book may be depressing you. If it is, that may be good as you will have something to practice with. I want you to focus on something that makes you feel down for about three minutes. Then begin reading the next paragraph.

Sit quietly with this feeling you have. Breathe in and out and feel the sensation in your body. Follow it wherever it takes you. Maybe it is in your chest, or your head, or even your belly. Do not judge it, or push it away. Just observe it. If you start to think of other things besides the sad or heavy feeling, come back to your breath and refocus on the original thought and feeling. Do this for about ten minutes and then start the next paragraph.

What you should be getting out of this is the realization that you are not your depression. The emotion depression, or any other emotion for that matter, is just like a coat you put on and off. If you can really get this concept and stay cognizant of it you may be able to prevent yourself from slipping into a deep depression. As always if you feel you are in danger of being clinically depressed you should seek the advice of a doctor. Whatever method you use to deal with depression is fine as long as you deal with it, and this meditation can be used with them. Remember you are not trying to push the depression away, just be with it. Yes, you are being compassionate with yourself once again. I have left some space on the page for your to record any thoughts on this meditation.

_____
_____
_____
_____
_____
_____
_____
_____
_____
_____
_____
_____
_____
_____
_____
_____
_____
_____
_____
_____
_____
_____

May 1st
(Two Weeks Later and No May Pole Dancing)

May Day, and here I sit with my foot up, no May pole dancing for this girl. One of my worst fears happened yesterday afternoon. I was getting out of my truck and I twisted my ankle, and fell on the pavement. Well nothing broke, and good for me I have my bone doctor appointment tomorrow, so while I am continuing the saga of the arthritis visit he can also look at my foot—ye ha!

I was going to wait until after my visit to share more of the journey, however while working in the garden this past weekend, I felt implored to add a few tidbits. I couldn't do much really, as I can't use my left index finger for pulling or for any labor activity without it swelling up and hurting. It was nice to get out in the courtyard though, and I did manage to plant two tomato plants. Gardening was my mother's legacy to me. She had the greenest thumb I ever saw, and as a small child I followed her around the garden all the time. She would send flowers to school with me for the teacher. This was the time I was most close to my mother, she was somewhat at peace in the yard, dabbling about with this or that project. I used to pick weeds and pretend I was cooking some magnificent dish.

I have a ponytail palm on the back porch. I placed some of her ashes and a picture of her raking in its' container. In the picture she is wearing a bubba hat with a big grin on her face. I picked up the picture and danced her around. Is she in the garden with us?

Testing
(A Patient's Experience)

Today is June 19; so much has happened in the past six-plus weeks. I have had five doctor visits, and been on two medications. Let us not forget the MRI of my neck that makes six. Also my aunt died. I want you to walk through all these experiences with me, for by now if you hadn't already figured it out, I need you. I need you to know how I really feel, and somehow in the telling perhaps I can ease your pain, whatever it may be. I don't even know who you are, but I feel you here as if you were reading these words as I form them, and place them on the paper. Hidden within the commitment to really share this with the world is an intimacy I have not felt before. Not only have I discovered my mothers' lost love, I have also made myself open to "people" as well. You people. I have not been willing to do that on this level before. Yes, I have read poetry and other items to people, but not written to people I have never met. I can almost feel you out there, and a desire is welling up in me, the desire to help you if I can. I feel a compassion I have read about, and tried to attain in Buddhist practice, but I don't think I ever really felt it spontaneously like this before. The only way I can really help you to heal is to share my own pain, my own revelation and affirm that somehow it can be a salve, or a spark, something positive for you. I am no Shaman, no Medicine Woman no spiritual Master. I am just a woman, trying to save herself from going mad, from becoming paralyzed or losing the muscle in her hand.

I want to live in usefulness, in joy, and touch those I love with a gentle gesture. Well that was a rush. My hands are tired, so I will close for now. Goodnight. Sleep well, my friends.

July 4th
(Reflecting on Family)

Independence Day, Webster says, "Independent—not subject to others, self reliant; free; valid in itself; politically of no party; Independence—being independent; self-reliance; self-support," "Day—period of 24 hours; time or unit of time; daylight; part of day occupied by certain activity; time period; special or designated day."

A time for self-reliance, a day designated to recognize the roots of our Country. Immigrants that did not want to be subject to others, that wanted to be free. These are my ancestors, and yours. There blood runs through our veins, there struggles are passed down through family patterns. Their toughness is in our bones. Today is really July 4, 2003 and I have not been feeling very self-reliant as my hand goes numb, and my shoulder seizes up. Perhaps I can find strength as I reflect on my ancestors. Perhaps you can find strength in yours.

My aunt that died last month was independent to the end. She was the glue that kept my father's side of the family together, a beautiful, strong compassionate woman. She was my godmother. My parents picked well, for she epitomized unconditional love, the kind of love god has for us. I loved her very much, and it speared my heart when she died, before I got a chance to see her. I had been planning to visit this year. I had a deep yearning to see the person I knew loved me, and looked like me, and to let her know how much I loved her.

Time waits for no one's good intentions. The family tree keeps expanding and it is up to you what kind of roots you weave. For the past two years I had tried to find the paper my aunt had written for me, with my family history. Last week I looked in a box determined to find

16

it. I found two letters from her, and then I found the paper. I put my family tree together on the computer. I was amazed at how big it seemed, compared to the view I had that my family was small. Granted, most of the people are deceased, but still I felt enveloped in this web. Who knows if these people would have loved me or not, but they are part of my heritage. I can't help but believe my aunt guided me to this discovery. I do not have any children, so in a sense, this book is my child that I pass down to you. If it helps you in your life then those changes and choices are like my grandchildren. Know that I love you, and them, and that you are part of a strong-willed, creative family.

I have been feeling weak dealing with pain, and my conditions. In looking back over my family history I feel more like an old salt, clawing my way through the hull of a sunken ship. This is a more heroic view. This Independence Day I choose to focus on the self-reliant person I have always been, keeping in mind that others have gone before with my burdens, and many others. When the fireworks go off tonight, I can imagine they are a sign to my ancestors that I am alive, and well in spirit, no matter what is going on in my body! Happy 4ᵗʰ of July.

Meditation on Others

This is not so much a meditation as it is recognition. As I am writing a journal entry I often break form and address you. This method may be unconventional to some, but to me it expresses my sincere effort to include you in my experience. I am writing this piece for you. I am hoping that if you identify with my experience and go where most people are afraid to go; into the heart of pain and suffering, that you will come out the other side less alone.

I want you to think of all the people that suffer as you do with pain. Be aware that many people have this disease, arthritis. It is a sad thought, but it can also be a joyful one. If you can help someone to feel comforted because you can identify with their physical and emotional pain, you have done a lot. I am not talking about commiserating. I am talking about recognizing them. People are generally afraid of pain and disability. They do not want it, or to be reminded of it. This causes many people to feel lost, alone, abandoned and in more pain. If you stop avoiding your own and other people's pain, there is a possibility it will lessen.

There is a seed of joy in what I just said. I am challenging you to step out of the stereotype of a "pain leper, "and into the role of an engaged compassionate being. What is that? It is a human being who cares as much about themselves as others. If you think I am assuming you are a terrible person, or a dolt, well I'm not. I just think that we all, myself Included, could reach out more. If you take the time to help someone that suffers in the same way you do, it can take the focus off your own pain and perhaps put a smile on their face.

I would like you to take some time to sit and think of all the people in your life that could use some cheering up. They could be family or friends. Perhaps it is someone you don't even know, or perhaps a co-worker. I am going to leave some space below for you to record the names of the people you think of, and to jot down an idea or two about how you could help them. They don't need to be someone who has a disability or are in physical pain. Whoever they are, they will be blessed by you for just thinking of helping them.

_____

_____

_____

_____

_____

_____

_____

_____

_____

_____

_____

_____

_____

_____

_____

_____

_____

_____

_____

_____

_____

_____

_____

_____

_____

_____

_____

October 10th
(Three Months Later)

Wow, I can't believe it is the end of the first week of October; where did the time go? Three months. I like the number 3, always have, however I did not mean for so much time to pass before I wrote again about this journey I am on. That being said let me catch you up.

I have been on several medications which at first seemed to help allay the pain in my joints, notwithstanding the side effects; much to my dismay, the relief from pain was only temporary, and I stopped taking the medication altogether. At first I was angry that modern medicine was not able to free me from constant irritation, and bouts of agony, especially when I moved into an apartment with stairs, and my knees, which had been two joints that had not haunted me, began to make it almost impossible to walk some days. Well, after the hurricanes at sea passed, the knee pain did also. So, now I am a meteorologist of sorts, a predictor of turbulence, and possible mayhem. Yes, this pain is much like a deadly storm, no matter how much you prepare for it, if it decides to make a direct hit, all you can do is endure.

Oh please, you say, enough with the clichés, and comparisons, take some aspirin and shut up. I know this is what some people think, those that have no idea what constant pain is like. I really don't care what they think because this book is not for them. I would hope to think it is for those people that have learned to endure, and yet still have hope of finding some type of cure, besides a barrel in the mouth, or some other method of permanent pain relief. I have never been one to run from a challenge, so no worry about PPR (permanent pain relief).

Sounds like I am rambling, so I will get to the points that lead me to begin writing again after three months. I decided to not take anymore prescriptions for this pain, at least for now, and intend on telling the neurologist this on my visit on Wednesday. I feel better mentally, and since moving, in spite of the knee problem, I have walked my dog twice a day around the new complex, have been on a modified Atkins diet, and began reading more about Tibetan Medicine (I practice Tibetan Buddhism). I have lost 9 pounds, something I was not able to do on the medication that was supposed to have a side effect of weight loss. There is a renewed optimism within my mind, and body. It hearkens back to my days in Santa Fe New Mexico in my late twenties when I totally believed in Alternative Medicine. It's not that I ever stopped; I just picked up a more rounded view with age. My view is this—whatever combination that works. So I am meditating every day, and doing other specific practices to assist my body, mind and spirit to work together. The goal is not necessarily to be free from pain although that would be great. The goal, if there is one is to be more balanced, more present, to enjoy each moment, hour day…that I live; to be more whole, to be compassionate to myself and others. Pain is not the enemy that I must kill with an operation or a pill. It is an organic part of my body/mind continuum, the result of thoughts and actions previous to the onset.

As I approach 50, and in the condition I am it occurs to me I have a choice. I can become an elderly person with a cabinet full of pills, and head for the grave smelling of aspercream, or…Those two letters, that one word, or…choice is born of that word. Well the choice is this. I can become an explorer, a cool gray haired Elder that has tasted her own marrow, and learned to live with it. There it is you guessed it, a splinterbone woman, master of her body, mind, and emotion, on a journey to the next great adventure whenever it comes. Living with pain as a companion if she needs to, ready to let that friend go if possible. Yes the goal is to continue on the journey, learning, growing, loving and transforming whatever she can.

This woman wears blue jeans, a cotton shirt, a vest, hiking boots, and a safari hat. She has a big smile on her sun beaten face. Sometimes she walks fast, sometimes slow with a walking stick. She loves to gaze at the moon and stars, to sleep out under the night sky, but not on the ground of course, because she loves her bones. She shares her journey with anyone who wants to come along. She thrills at new places, those tender, powerful spots in nature that swallow you up, and give you back to yourself whole. This woman's journey will never end no matter if she dies tomorrow, or lives well on into her hundreds. Even after she is gone from this Earth in form, she will come back again, and again, to lead others on the journey to the center of themselves. She is a Buddhist; she aspires to be a Bodhisattva, a being of compassion, leading other s out of suffering, until none are left to suffer.

This is what I am. So, I give to you the truth, that at the core of your pain, whatever kind it may be, is a splinterbone woman, a being of great compassion, and a warrior woman that can look at pain, and both spit in its face, and cuddle it like a hurt child. Yes, whatever it takes. That is medicine, alternative, or otherwise.

December 27th
(After Christmas)

A lot has happened in the past two months. In October it appears there was a lot of focus on "I", and perhaps into November, as" I" started a master's program. Perhaps this is where a lot of pain comes from, focusing on one's self, or one's image of self. In any case Christmas has come and gone, pain has returned, a close friend has cancer, and life marches on.

This Christmas Eve, I stayed at my sister's house. I was able to do this without resentment, or overwhelming sadness. I was able to look at pictures of family, and find papers with my mother's history, along with a letter describing her childhood tragedies. The point I am making is the season is about focusing on others, giving to others. This is the message of Jesus and Buddha. This is the true key to being pain free. Drugs can come and go, alternative medicine can come and go, and true giving can set you free.

Oh sure you say, it is the Holiday Season, a few months ago it was Tibetan Medicine going to free her, and now it is the spirit of Christmas, oh boy. You may be right; I may not be able to hold onto the essence of truth discovered, and carry it forth into the New Year. You probably think I will make some fantastic resolution, but I think not. If I have learned anything in December it is that life is unpredictable, time rushes on, and the moment, whether it is filled with joint pain, or any other kind, is the only moment we have.

I had planned to finish this book in February when my niece has her baby. She is due February 14 the day after my mother's three-year anniversary of her passing. The baby's name is Alexandra, the first and maybe only great-granddaughter of my mother. My niece has had a difficult pregnancy, and surely has endured a lot of pain in one form or another, and will when the baby is born. This brings me back to the theme of this month, forgetting one's own pain for the sake of others. That is what a mother does when she gives birth. She endures for her child. She splits her pelvis bones, so the child can enter the world. She becomes a splinterbone woman at that moment.

My niece looks more and more like my mother the older she gets, and in looking at pictures of my grandmother and great-grandmother, I also see the resemblance. I do not know what Alexandra will look like, but I am sure she will carry with her the history of my mother, and will become a splinterbone woman herself. She will be fiercely independent, strong, speak her mind, and have a fantastic sense of humor. She will have opportunities my mother only imagined in her wildest dreams. I pray she does not have the physical ailments I or my sister has, but whatever life has in store for her, I know she will be loved by all those around her, and that my mother wherever she is will look over her.

December 28th
(Reflecting the Next Day)

When the world is quiet, and the clouds are hung grey, and low, there is a stillness that takes over my being. The hawks glide on the thermals, and I am reminded of a time when I was young, and wandered the woods of my hometown. In nature everything made sense. There was no sense of false striving, a mad spin to nowhere. Effort was purposeful, practical, and all acts lead to fulfillment. If you took a hike it was to get somewhere, and enjoy the view.

Tomorrow is Monday, and as I imagine my return to work, it feels like a solid wall of endless activity. Like a machine marching on consuming whatever is in its way. Where am I going with this? Well I am acutely aware of the passage of time reflected in my aging face, and the quick growth of my young nephews. It causes me to ponder what is important to complete before my bones too are splintered, and ground into a fine powder. I twirl around in my head the desire to create a great work, and it bounces off the stillness and simplicity of those clouds sitting in the sky. My views on impermanence spur me on to complete what I need to, and at the same time, the knowledge that everything is impermanent says, why strive?

I could sit for days, and just feel those clouds's and watch the lake beneath them ripple, and glitter, and what would be wrong with that? My mother would say I was thinking too much, or wasting time, being lazy. What she would have me do, I can only speculate. Always, I am trying to figure out the best course to follow, oh you too? Do I pull my old business ideas out, and rejuvenate them, or perhaps I should let them go and do something different, yet similar?

I want to benefit beings, and leave a legacy for my young niece, and nephews. I want them to be able to draw strength from my struggle, and those of my forbearers. I want to leave the planet with something that will help them find a way to peace, and healing while alive, and to find enlightenment.

Sometimes I just want to be a monk in an empty room with a cushion, and maybe a few good books. No clutter, no lists, no deadlines. There are so many books now on making life simple, and that is not what this one is about; however, you can't help but touch on the topic when you are considering the effects your mother's death has on you, or anyone else's for that matter. You always think of the things you would have said or done if you had had more time with them, and how insignificant a lot of our activity is in the face of death.

January 12th
(After the Sage Speaks)

Last night I listened to one of the lamas from the monastery speak. The topic was on finding happiness within this life of impermanence. It was like a breath of fresh air to hear him talk about not finding happiness in external things, that whatever we do with our talent, and life, we should benefit beings. I know this simple yet difficult truth. No matter what you do, be compassionate to yourself, and others. Perhaps that is the problem I have been having. Maybe I have not been compassionate to myself in not wanting to be self centered; perhaps I have been too driven to do something. I don't really know. I do know I am in a lot of physical pain again with this weather. Menopause is really hitting hard also. I feel like drinking, and crawling out of my skin. I feel like I will just go nuts if I do not do something creative, instead of push papers in a little closed up room called my job.

As you see, I am falling into the illusion that if the pain stops or I "figure out something," everything will be "ok." In other words, if I am out of pain, and figure out a solution to my mind numbing job, "fixing those external things" will make me happy or at peace, or something. This is just what the Lama was talking about. No accomplishment or circumstance is going to fix things, and make me happy. Even if the pain stops, and I sell this book, and never had to work again; life would change, externals would change, and something else would disrupt the illusion of okay ness. I think I am doing battle with my own illusory mind, and am blaming arthritis, and menopause. Granted those things are not helping matters, but they are not really the cause of the root pain.

Aha! Could it be my mother's circumstances, tragic though they were, were not the root cause of her pain? Could this be true for all of you also? Could I, she, and you be ok just the way we are, and yet still have room to clear away the debris? It sounds so simple, yet, time and time again, as you can see by reading all I have written, I get constantly caught up with the need to figure things out, to make things be a certain way so I will be alright. Sometimes I just think I have attention deficit disorder, who knows perhaps I do, but I think it is clear the goose chase is on whether I do, or I don't.

I think the revelation is this. Stop seeking. Cease and desist looking for an answer to the pain, confusion, and right course of action, for the pain, or my great life's work. What would happen if I, you, and everyone else stopped? Let's try it right now. Just stop reading. Sit and close your eyes, still your mind and be...What happened? Well for me, I had an overwhelming feeling like I needed to protect myself, that if I did not do something, then something...would happen. Perhaps this is just paranoia. I rather think it is an effect of the rat race mentality. Everything is moving so fast, if I stop I will get passed up, passed by and lose...

Are you afraid to be ordinary? Are you reading this book looking to somehow feel better about yourself, and be more? Well I hope you do feel better, and we are all ordinary, and extraordinary, and both are ok. Hmmm, I say this to feel safe. I learned it. How do I really feel? How do you really feel? Are you getting uncomfortable reading this, do you want me to stop? Do you want me to shut up, and say something profound, or flowery? I am going to stop, and take the dog out, as she feels the need to go, and be in the moment.

February 4th
(Three Weeks Waiting)

That was a long walk, wasn't it? Do you see how life comes along, and just sweeps you up? I never got back here on that day three weeks ago. A lot has happened in three weeks. My niece's grandfather passed away a little over a week ago. He was a wonderful man, kind, compassionate, a real leader. We will all miss him greatly.

The baby is not here yet, but will be soon. We await her, and look to her to bring new life into the family, with her smiling face, and purity. My mothers' birthday was two days ago. My sister and I thought, perhaps the baby would come on that day, and that my mother may come back through her. Now, I see that was a silly thought. I think my mother has gone on a long time ago, and that this baby, whoever she was in a past life, will be an independent being. Next week will be the anniversary of my mother's death. It will have been three years ago. It will also be a year ago that I started this book. What have I learned in a year? How have I changed?

I am more at peace with my mother. I deal better with the pain of my maladies. They have taken their toll though when it comes to fatigue, and stress. I do not have stress under control, and don't know if I ever will. I have learned to be more compassionate, and to let things go. My relationship with my sister is better. As I made peace with my mother, and accepted her, I have made peace in my own mind, with my sister as well. I will never get from people what I really want, and need. Once this is accepted across the board, then there will be no disappointment, no yearning, and seeking. I see that this is also the solution to my stress at work. Expect nothing. Create a better future for myself, yes, but expect nothing from them. Drop blame, and focus on what is in front of you. I think all my anger and frustration comes from wanting things to be different, whether it is justified or not. I need to accept things as they are, and move on. It doesn't sound very heroic. This is the stable side of being a splinterbone woman; sitting down in the dirt with oneself, and becoming an immovable force of acceptance. Let them come at me with their demands and deadlines. I will draw inside the blanket of the moment, and feel the journey beneath. When I look up, and into their eyes, whatever the pressing need is, will seem insignificant. The medicine of the moment, the remedy, will reveal itself. Instead of clinching my jaw, and feeling overwhelmed, I will have a mountain top moment in the middle of an audit. I will watch the dance, and sit in the dirt, an old splinterbone woman that people scoff at. Look at her dirty old blanket they will say. She stares at nothing, and has a silly grin on her lips, what is she thinking? I will be thinking nothing. I will be at peace in the moment, wrapped in wisdom. I will not expect them to respect this wisdom blanket—no I will not. I will send out thoughts of love, and compassion, because they need it more than I.

Meditation on Mindfulness

I would like to take a moment to talk to you about mindfulness. Mindfulness is about staying totally aware of everything in and around you. It is like a meditation in motion. It is another tool to stay focused in the present instead of caught up in pain, or whatever chaos may be going on in your mind or immediate environment. First I will give you an example of how to practice mindfulness, and then you will get a chance to do it.

Let's say you are sitting in your living room. You would begin by being aware of your breath, how it felt going in and out of your nose, how your chest rises and falls. You then could focus on feeling where your body connects to the chair, your back, legs, bottom, arms, and feet on the floor. You could then look around you, not thinking about anything in particular, just observing. If thoughts come in, just let them flow by. If you get up and move around the room you would focus on each step as each part of your foot contacts the floor. I think you probably have the idea now how this works.

Why would you want to do this? The purpose is to be totally in the present, not judging your surroundings. It has many benefits. For one, you are totally present in your body, and this helps create balance on a physical level. If you practice this kind of mindfulness all day you would find you are more in control of your emotions and actions. Being mindful gives you that extra second or two to think, when you are in a conversation with someone. I would like you to practice mindfulness for about fifteen to twenty minutes in an undisturbed area and write about the experience. If it is a positive tool for you great, if not that is okay too.

Alexandra
(She is Finally Here)

"I look into your searching eyes, upon your beautiful perfect face and see delight. Your parents are awed at your arrival. Your mother is a fierce lioness, your father a tender proud man. This is the moment I have been waiting for, the birth of the next splinterbone woman. I bless you with a Buddhist prayer, and tell you that I love you." Well now you all know that my great-niece Alexandra is here. She arrived February 15, two days after the 3 year anniversary of my mother's passing. It has been a year since I began this book, and I have been waiting for her birth to wrap it up.

It seems like a new chapter should begin with the birth of Alexandra, and she may be the topic of another story at another time. I want to let her be, to make her own way without my commentary. I will talk about how she impacts me though. She reminds me that we all come into this world with a fresh start. Even if you believe in reincarnation, and that you bring past karma with you, it still is a fresh start with a new body, and new opportunities to be a pure light upon this planet. I think she is off to a good start with her parents. I imagine my parents as infants. They came into the world full of promise. Their parents looked upon them with the same delight, wondering what they could, or would become, hoping for the best. The thing I want to take away most from that first view is that wise innocence we all have that first day we were born. We breathed for the first time, felt the air against our skin, and had our first meal and our first fart. Our elders looked upon us without judgment, looked only for the good, for the potential.

Fresh new skin, clear eyes, all the attributes of a creature growing and thriving.

This first day of life, this ecstatic moment is the seed of spirituality. We are set on a path that day, a path to find out who we are. It is clear to me now that we arrive as who we are; a beautiful flower bud waiting to bloom, a fully formed miracle here to delight, and create joy for those around us. The challenge is to stay mindful of that as the years pass, as problems come and go, as the body ages, and creates splinters in our bones.

March 1st
(A Year Later)

It feels like spring today as I sit here on the back porch looking at the lake. Birds are all about making nests, singing their hearts out. Kids are playing on the grass, and Lulu my dog watches it all, wishing she could run, and chase everything in sight. Last night we saw an otter in the back lake. It rose right up out of the water, and looked at us. It reminded me of all the wild creatures in the woods, and the wild creature within me. Spring does that, makes you want to run, and jump, and frolic. Today my knee is out again so I can't do any frolicking. Soon I will have to get it checked out, and fixed if necessary.

I don't want to go into a diatribe about pain, or sorrow about my body falling apart. I want to finish this book as a splinterbone woman. I want to dig deep, and give you something that will give you hope, and strength, and inspiration. I am going to do a meditation on the lake, and see what it has to say, and share that with you.

Her surface has many faces. Sometimes clear, and still as glass, she reflects the sky, and shore around her, but then the slightest bit of breeze, and her mood changes with ripples, wrinkling her wide smile. If rain comes she gets choppy, and does a dance with the sky water. The one thing that remains consistent about her though, is her depth. You cannot see into her, whatever secrets she has, remain hidden beneath, no matter how changeable she may be on the surface. The mystery of her bottom water makes me feel anchored, and secure, like she could hold all my pain, and just fill up on it without loosing anything.

This brings to mind the Tibetan practice of sending and receiving. In a nutshell this means you think of someone who needs healing, or has hurt you, and you breathe in all the pain, imagining it as black smoke. You then breathe out white light to the person, healing them. You become a transformer of pain. The lake does this for me as I gaze at her, and let go my sorrow. I come away with the joy of watching her glisten, and dance with the wind. Nature is a great healer. So what does she say to you? She says come, and sit by my shore, dip your feet in if you can, and feel the cool liquid. Let your bones float upon my surface; I will support you if you let me. Be as a little child again, for in those moments of surrender, you will find strength. Visit me often, for the world can be a harsh place. You cannot cross a desert without sufficient water, nor can you function in the modern world without the balance of nature, and her solace. I am here for you; all I ask is that you keep me clean so I can care for the creatures that share my body. They will help you too, if you let them. The fishes, turtles, otters, birds, even the grasses that rise up around me.

Funny, the reason the body breaks down in the first place is due to being out of balance. It seems I need to take the advice of the Lake as well. A reprioritization is in store. I used to take time every year to reread my journals, and take stock of the cycles of change I had gone through, and would get a new bearing on the course of my life. I would see how I had grown in some areas, and how some things seemed to stay the same. I have gotten away from this over the past number of years. I think leading the professional, stable life, while it has had its benefits, has robbed me of a certain kind of wisdom. My claws have dulled. So the question is how can they be sharpened without throwing out the stability?

It is clear that one must continually re-craft their life to stay on a path of growth and sanity. It does not really matter what motivates you. If having a painful body does it, great, or if it is a death of someone close, great. Whatever the reason, acknowledge the gift, and begin the renovation. Are you inspired yet? Remember I said I wanted to end this book by inspiring you. When you read the last page, I want you to be able to say, "Wow, I really got something out of that that I can actually use." I want you to be able to come back to this book and find yourself again if you get lost. I want you to remember that you can start your day, or life, over at any moment. I want you to remember to sit by the lake, or under a tree, or by the ocean, or anywhere in nature, and talk to her, listen to her, and find your center.

I am reminded of the time I was hiking in the Haleakala Crater on the Island of Maui, Hawaii. I was on a self proclaimed vision quest. All I had was a small bag, and the clothes on my back. No money, or food, and a small amount of water. As I walked in the hot sun, there was not a sound to be heard, except the molecules bouncing off each other. As I watched every step, as the path was full of razor-sharp lava rock, a message came to me. It said, put one foot in front of the other, and focus on the path in front of you. Trust that I will lead you. Trust who? You can interpret that however you want. The point is, to stay focused, or mindful, of what you are doing each moment. I know I have said this many times already, but it warrants repeating, as it is so hard to stay that focused, and not get caught up in our lives, and all its problems.

I am telling you to take the time to find the magic in the moment, no matter what is going on in your body, or life, at the moment. Be a splinterbone woman. Be the explorer, the medicine woman, the healer, whatever you want to call yourself. Take off the label your pain, or malady has put on you, and be the wild creature, or the mellow creature sitting by the lake. Burrow deep down inside yourself, and listen to the ancient one. Listen to your ancestors, all those women that came before you. Remember their names, call them out. Ask them to gather round you for council. Put your problems before them, and listen to what they tell you.

Can you imagine a room full of the women from your line, generation after generation of strong women, splinterbone women, with such stories to tell? They have endured much pain, and I am sure they danced the dance of joy a time or two. Call on them to help you through. Their essence is yours, their bones are within you.

This is a fitting end to this book, a gathering of my female ancestors. Yes, I will have this gathering, and tell you about it. I will ask them if they have a special message for my readers. Now, I am excited, and a little nervous, but alive, yes, alive with spring in my veins. It is the true me, the one who dances under the full moon, a wild splinterbone woman. I am really getting close now, close to the end of this book, and close to its birth, and I get to have all the women of my line there with me. Now I must prepare.

The Message
(This Is Mine; Discover Yours)

Know that my body is yours, that we fill up every particle, every space of being. Solid as a rock, and empty as space, we are one. Sit in that solidity, and draw strength from the silence, feel us course through your veins, the life blood of all women, from all times. The earth is in the belly of our being, of our consciousness. We created her from the dust of our bones, the bones of all women. We have toiled, and endured, so you may have life, so you may plant the green things upon her, and water them with your dreams, with your visions of what joy can be. You are a creative force and a receptacle all at the same time. Do not be afraid of this truth, this power. You are here to create, protect what you create, and let it go, to recreate. So it has always been, and forever shall be. We smile upon you, and we are within your very bones, feel us, we are all one. Words could not say more.

This is what is said through me. I could not prepare for this, I tried, but to no avail. I woke up hours ago on this March 7th full moon morning. I could not sleep, and began to think of all my ancestors. They just kept growing, and growing, in number, and they filled the room with their presence, I imagined they were little girls, wise, yet youthful creatures, so ancient, and yet fresh as spring, innocent. I let their presence fill my body, could feel the heat move through my hands, and strength, fill my entire body. I sit here now, writing this, sensing a state of mind beyond fear, beyond pain, beyond all the suffering of all those women. It is almost indescribable. It is a feeling of completion, a warm, soothing, peacefulness. It is like the end of a journey, and also the beginning.

My personal struggles with religion, spirituality, gender inequality, and every other struggle I have had, seem to melt away within this inner space. This is my truth, my experience, and I do not have to convince anyone of it. I share it, for that is what my path is, to share my walk. If you want to walk with me great, if not, that is fine too. I have to say that the sense of urgency to do something melts away within this experience. I have sought this solid feeling, and could not find it. I danced with the children of my ancestors, and it came upon me. You know bones appear solid, and yet, they are organic growing material. When the flesh melts off of them, they really seem solid, and yet they are porous, and the wind can play a melody through them. Time hollows out the space where lyrics emerge from. These words are the truth of the ages, the witness to the laws of nature spoken freely.

Each of us has a song within our bones, ultimately the same message, but told in a different way. Each chord makes up a chorus, called diversity. May the women of the world sing together, and teach their children to do so also. May prejudice fade, and be not heard above this rhapsody.

Yesterday I went to the Indian Festival. There were not many vendors there, but it still made me cry to hear the drumming, to feel the rhythm of my ancestors. I felt my father was there, I imagined we were in Indian dress dancing. My mother was always at odds with that part of his heritage. This has always made me feel sad, and torn, not really belonging to any race, or culture. The experience I have just had with my ancestors brings peace. I now know my mother has moved beyond her prejudice. Each race is a part of the melody. All the songs are within me, and this splinterbone woman is not afraid to say that.

I think of Alexandra, my great—niece; now she is a beautiful mix of cultures. She has a strong line of women behind her, within her. I want her to learn how powerful she is, and not take on the trappings of this world, and its ignorance of woman power. She will find her own way of course, as will all of you. I do want her, and you to know what lies within you. I want you to take the time to sit with yourself, and find the wisdom within your bones. Go out and sit upon the earth, feel her strength move up your spine. Cry into her, bleed into her. I promise you it will not be a fruitless experience, if you give it half a chance. Some day your bones will return to her, weather whole, or as dust. If you sit with her now, this truth will not scare you as much, or perhaps at all.

I will share a story of a time when I sat on the earth in this way. I was living in the mountains of New Mexico. I was living outside, and this particular day, I had my period. I used to suffer from extreme cramps that nothing would stop. I created a circle, and I had a large tree root in the center. I put all sorts of objects upon it that meant something to me. By this time it was getting dark, and the mists were gathering. It was cold, but I had a blanket. That is all I had on, a blanket. I sat on the earth, and bled into her. I sang, and cried, and rocked, and probably looked quite crazy, but I did not care. I drew strength from the earth, from the experience. It was a raw feeling sitting there, half naked in the mist, with darkness all around, just me, and the planet. Perhaps this sounds a bit extreme, or perhaps not, but stripping oneself down physically, mentally, and emotionally, has a way of cleansing, and rebuilding one.

This was a real moment, nothing like television, or even film, or even like reading this, or any other book. This was a deeply personal experience. This was something a splinterbone woman would do. My mother probably never sat naked on a mountain top to bleed, but I am sure in essence, she had similar experiences, and my other ancestors did as well. If I had all their stories, what a tale that would tell, so the next thing I am going to suggest to you, is to take the time to talk to all the women in your family, and get those stories, if they are willing to tell them. Write them down, tape them, and capture them in some fashion, for they are a priceless gift. They are Herstory!

When the day is done, and the television is off, and the bills have been paid, and all your *stuff* has been secured for the night, what are you left with? Your family, if they are with you, and yourself. Yes, and your ancestors, and all their adventures. How much more interesting is that than a sitcom? Think about it, and how you are spending your time. That is all I am going to say about that.

I sit here looking at this page, knowing I am at the end. My bone saga continues. On Monday I get the results of an MRI of my knee. Hopefully, I will not need surgery, but if I do, I will have all my ancestors there with me to help endure. I was not going to end this piece with talk of pain, and suffering, but that is how this all began; with my mothers death, and being cast in her osteo image. It has been a long journey, and yet, this past year has flown by so quickly. All the same rituals are occurring in this tourist haven, yet I, am not the same.

Each day I get older, and feel like my body falls apart more rapidly, but the paradox is, that I am made more whole because of it. I am rebuilt on the inside, if I allow it to happen. This is the gift I leave you with, the realization that even though we are in an impermanent existence, the wisdom gained is indestructible.

About the Author

Laura Folk currently works in the Social Services field. She is also a Massage Therapist, Polarity Therapist, Reiki Practitioner, Universal Life Minister, a Poet. She was born in New Jersey, has lived in Santa Fe, New Mexico, Hawaii, and currently lives in Florida. This is her first book

0-595-31647-6

www.ingramcontent.com/pod-product-compliance
Lightning Source LLC
Chambersburg PA
CBHW021303280526
45784CB00005B/2495